If I Was A Man

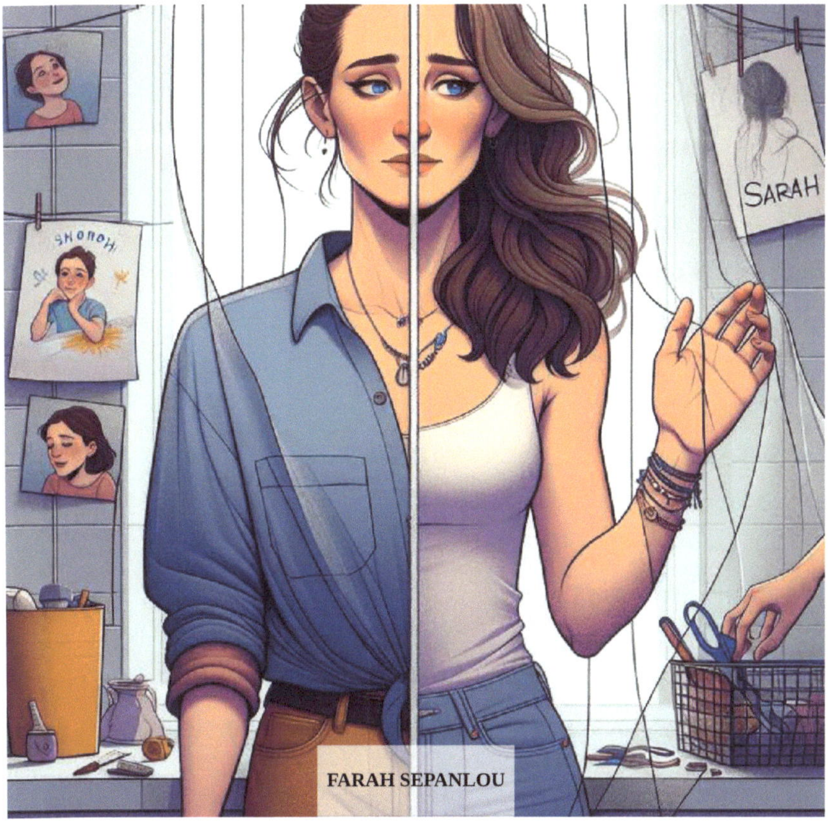

FARAH SEPANLOU

SUMMARY

Chapter 1: Awakening to a New Reality — 2

1.1 Sarah's startling discovery — 2

1.2 Confusion and denial — 4

1.3 Seeking answers — 6

Chapter 2: Facing the World — 9

2.1 First steps into the unknown — 9

2.2 Encountering disbelief — 11

2.3 The struggle for acceptance — 13

Chapter 3: The Quest for Identity — 16

3.1 Exploring a dual existence — 16

3.2 Confronting inner turmoil — 16

3.3 Embracing change — 16

Chapter 4: Trials and Tribulations — 22

4.1 Navigating societal norms — 22

4.2 Bonds tested and broken — 24

4.3 Finding allies in unexpected places — 25

Chapter 5: The Search for Resolution — 28

5.1 A journey towards understanding — 28

5.2 Challenges of transformation — 30

5.3 Acceptance and the path forward — 32

Chapter 6: Embracing Change and Moving Forward — 35

6.1 Overcoming Fear and Resistance — 35

6.2 Finding Support and Building a Support System — 37

6.3 Setting Goals and Taking Action — 39

1

Awakening to a New Reality

1.1 Sarah's startling discovery

Sarah woke to the soft murmur of the city outside her window, a familiar yet always distant cacophony. The morning light spilled across her bed, casting shadows that danced with the rhythm of a world she felt increasingly alienated from. As she stretched, expecting the usual stiffness from nights spent curled around worries and regrets, she paused. Something was profoundly different.

"What in the world?" Sarah murmured to herself, disbelief coloring her tone as she discovered changes in her body that defied explanation. A physical manifestation of her fleeting wish to escape the burdens of her femininity had inexplicably become reality overnight.

Her mind raced with questions and fears as she tried to piece together how this could have happened. Was it a dream? A bizarre twist of fate? She reached for her phone, hesitating before dialing her best friend, Jamie.

"Jamie, you're not going to believe what's happened," Sarah started without preamble once the call connected.

"Try me," Jamie replied, a note of amusement in their voice that quickly turned into concern as Sarah recounted her morning discovery.

"This is...Sarah, are you sure? I mean, it sounds like something out of a sci-fi novel," Jamie said after a moment of stunned silence.

"I know how it sounds! But I'm telling you, it's real. I don't know what to do," Sarah confessed, the weight of confusion and fear pressing down on her.

"You're not alone in this, okay? We'll figure it out together," Jamie assured her firmly.

The conversation shifted as they brainstormed possible explanations and solutions. Hormonal imbalances? A medical anomaly? Nothing seemed to fit perfectly with Sarah's experience. Jamie suggested seeking medical advice but also offered unwavering support regardless of the outcome.

Gratitude washed over Sarah for having someone in her life who could offer such unconditional support despite the absurdity of the situation. Yet beneath that gratitude lay a roiling sea of emotions—fear, confusion, but also an undeniable curiosity about what this change might mean for her life moving forward.

1.2 Confusion and denial

Sarah's morning had unfolded into an afternoon of disbelief and denial. The world outside continued its usual pace, oblivious to the turmoil that had upended her reality. She found herself oscillating between a desperate attempt to rationalize her situation and a deep-seated fear of what it truly meant.

"It has to be some sort of mistake," Sarah muttered to herself, examining her reflection for the umpteenth time, hoping to find something she had missed. "Things like this just don't happen."

The sound of her phone ringing broke through her spiraling thoughts. It was Jamie again, checking in after their earlier conversation.

"Hey, how are you holding up?" Jamie's voice was laced with concern.

"I... I don't know," Sarah confessed, her voice barely above a whisper. "Part of me thinks I'm losing my mind."

"Listen, Sarah," Jamie said firmly. "You're not losing your mind. But maybe we should consider all possibilities—no matter how outlandish they seem."

Their conversation meandered through possibilities that seemed ripped from the pages of fantasy novels or the scripts of science fiction films. Each suggestion seemed more improbable than the last, but discussing them brought a strange comfort to Sarah.

"What if," Jamie hesitated, "what if this is something... supernatural? Or extraterrestrial?"

Despite the seriousness of their discussion, Sarah couldn't help but let out a short laugh. "Now we're entering conspiracy theory territory."

"Maybe so," Jamie conceded with a chuckle. "But until we have a better explanation, everything is on the table."

Their exchange did little to solve the mystery but provided Sarah with a much-needed distraction from her fears. As they said their goodbyes, promising to talk again soon, Sarah felt a sliver of hope amidst the confusion.

Yet as night fell and Sarah lay in bed once more, surrounded by silence rather than the comforting sounds of Jamie's theories, doubt crept back in. Was there truly an explanation for what had happened? Or was she alone in an experience beyond understanding?

In those quiet moments before sleep claimed her, Sarah realized that denial could only take her so far. Tomorrow would bring its own challenges and perhaps even answers—but for now, she allowed herself to drift off into a restless sleep filled with dreams that blurred the lines between reality and fantasy even further.

1.3 Seeking answers

The dawn brought with it a resolve in Sarah to seek out answers, no matter how elusive they might be. The morning air was crisp, filled with the scent of a world waking up, unaware of the turmoil within her. Today, she decided, would be different. Today, she would start looking for explanations.

"I need to understand what's happening," Sarah said to herself as she prepared for the day ahead. Her determination was palpable, a stark contrast to the confusion and denial that had plagued her just hours before.

Her first stop was the local library, a place she remembered fondly as a sanctuary of knowledge and discovery. As she walked through its familiar aisles, Sarah felt a sense of purpose guiding her steps.

"Can I help you find something?" asked Martha, the librarian who had known Sarah since she was a child.

"Yes, I'm looking for anything on... unusual phenomena," Sarah replied hesitantly, unsure of how much to reveal.

Martha raised an eyebrow but nodded understandingly. "Let's see what we can find." Together, they delved into old texts and modern articles alike, searching for anything that might shed light on Sarah's experience.

Their search was exhaustive but fruitless. "I'm sorry, dear," Martha finally said with a sigh. "It seems like what you're looking for doesn't want to be found."

Sarah felt a twinge of disappointment but thanked Martha for her help. As she left the library, her phone buzzed with a message from Jamie: "Meet me at the café? I think I found something."

Intrigued and hopeful, Sarah quickened her pace towards their meeting spot. Upon arrival, Jamie greeted her with an excited smile.

"You won't believe this," Jamie began without preamble. "I spoke to my cousin who works in astrophysics. He mentioned some classified research about anomalies similar to what you described."

"So there might actually be an explanation?" Sarah asked cautiously optimistic.

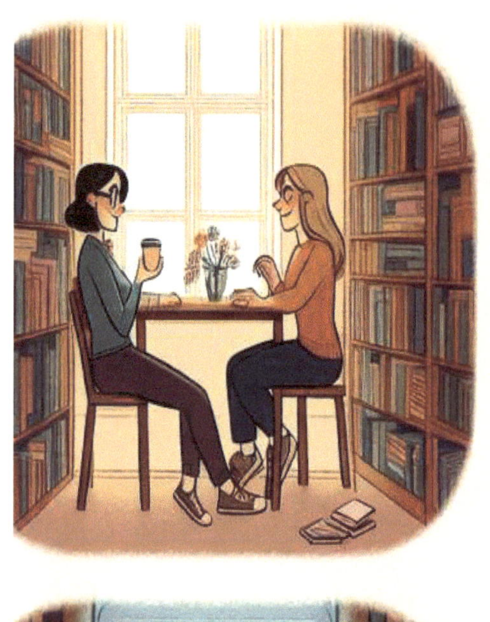
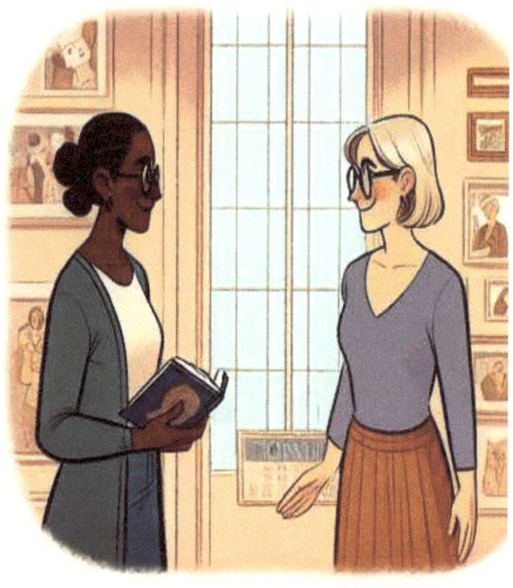
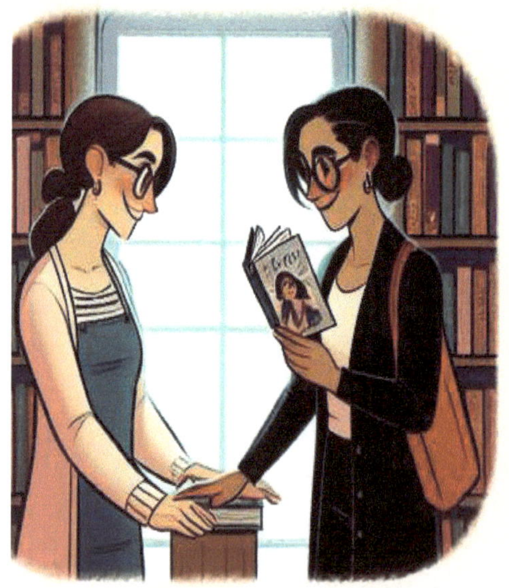
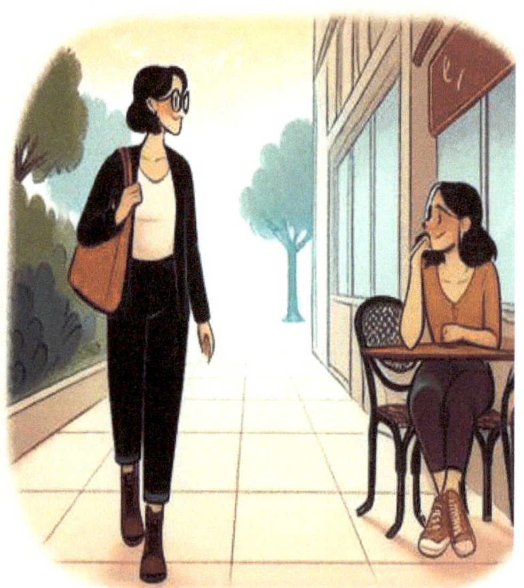

Sarah listened intently as Jamie recounted the conversation with his cousin. While it was all speculative and second-hand information, it opened up new avenues of thought and investigation that neither had considered before.

"Possibly," Jamie replied with a grin. "But we'll need to dig deeper."

As they discussed their next steps over coffee, Sarah felt a renewed sense of hope and determination. The path ahead was uncertain and likely fraught with challenges, but for the first time since this ordeal began, she believed that answers were within reach.

2

Facing the World

2.1 First steps into the unknown

Sarah, now grappling with an unexpected transformation, found herself at the threshold of a reality she had never imagined. The morning light did little to dispel the confusion and fear that had settled in her heart. As she navigated her new existence, the first challenge was confronting her own reflection—a stranger's gaze meeting hers in the mirror.

"How do I face the world?" Sarah whispered to her reflection, a question that seemed to echo back at her with no answer. The day demanded she step out into a world that had not changed as she had. Her first encounter was with her neighbor, Mrs. Thompson, who noticed something different but couldn't quite place it.

"Sarah? You look... different today," Mrs. Thompson remarked, squinting her eyes slightly.

"It's been a rough night," Sarah managed to say, her voice betraying a hint of its new depth.

The real test came when dropping off her children at school. Their acceptance was immediate and unquestioning; their love unconditional. "Daddy?" her youngest asked in confusion only once before accepting Sarah's explanation that sometimes change is outside our control but doesn't alter love.

Work presented its own set of challenges and revelations. Her colleagues reacted with varying degrees of surprise, discomfort, and curiosity. Yet, it was during a lunch break conversation that Sarah found an unexpected ally in Tom, a co-worker who had quietly navigated his own journey of self-discovery.

"You're not alone in feeling out of place," Tom confided after sharing his story, offering Sarah a glimpse of understanding and camaraderie she desperately needed.

This day marked Sarah's first steps into an unknown world—a world where every interaction was a negotiation between who she was, who she appeared to be now, and who she wanted to become. Despite the contradictions and challenges, these initial encounters sowed seeds of hope that perhaps understanding and acceptance were not as far off as they seemed.

2.2 Encountering disbelief

Sarah's journey into the unknown took a sharp turn as she encountered disbelief from those who had known her before. The skepticism wasn't just a barrier; it was a mirror reflecting the myriad doubts she harbored within herself. Each interaction became a tightrope walk between revealing her truth and protecting her heart from the harsh judgments of disbelief.

"But how can this be?" asked an old friend, his voice laced with incredulity. "People don't just change overnight." His words, meant to express confusion, felt like daggers to Sarah. She had hoped for support, but found herself needing to justify her existence.

"I know it's hard to understand," Sarah replied, her voice steady despite the turmoil inside. "I'm still me, just... different." Her attempt at explanation hung in the air, met with a silence that spoke volumes.

The disbelief wasn't confined to friends alone. Family gatherings became battlegrounds where whispered conversations and sideways glances were as tangible as the air she breathed. "It's just a phase," one relative muttered under their breath, not quiet enough for Sarah not to hear.

Yet, it was during these moments of doubt that Sarah found unexpected allies. Her sister, once distant, stepped forward with an open heart. "I don't fully understand," she admitted during a rare moment of vulnerability between them, "but I see you're still the person I love and respect."

This acknowledgment was a balm to Sarah's weary soul. It reminded her that while disbelief could be disheartening, it also offered an opportunity for dialogue—for breaking down barriers and building bridges of understanding.

As Sarah navigated through waves of skepticism and acceptance alike, she realized that encountering disbelief was not just about facing others' doubts but also about confronting her own fears. With each conversation, each look of confusion or acceptance, she grew stronger in her resolve to live authentically.

Through these trials by fire, Sarah learned an invaluable lesson: belief in oneself is the first step toward fostering understanding in others. And sometimes, the most profound changes come not from altering perceptions but from embracing one's truth amidst disbelief.

2.3 The struggle for acceptance

Sarah's journey of self-discovery and the quest for acceptance unfolded with each step she took into the world. Her path was fraught with challenges, each encounter a test of her resilience and determination to be understood and embraced for who she truly was.

"You're really going through with this?" her colleague Mark asked one afternoon, skepticism written all over his face. His question wasn't new to Sarah; it echoed the doubts of many around her.

"Yes, I am," Sarah responded, her voice a mixture of patience and weariness. "It's not about 'going through with something' as much as it is about being true to myself."

The workplace had become another arena where Sarah felt she had to constantly defend her identity. Conversations by the water cooler or during lunch breaks often veered into personal territories, leaving Sarah feeling exposed and vulnerable.

However, it was in these moments of vulnerability that unexpected gestures of support emerged. A quiet nod from Jenna, the receptionist, or a warm smile from Mr. Thompson in accounting became small beacons of hope. "I admire your courage," Jenna whispered one day, her words lifting Sarah's spirits more than she could have imagined.

Yet, acceptance was not universal. Some colleagues avoided eye contact, while others whispered behind closed doors. The divide between support and silence grew wider, but so did Sarah's resolve.

"Why do you think people struggle to accept change in others?" Sarah asked Jenna during a rare moment of quiet.

"Fear," Jenna replied after a thoughtful pause. "Fear of what they don't understand or can't predict."

This insight struck a chord with Sarah. She realized that her journey wasn't just about seeking acceptance from others but also about challenging their fears and preconceptions.

As days turned into weeks, Sarah found that small victories in acceptance were monumental. Each conversation that ended with understanding rather than judgment, every gesture of kindness over indifference, fortified her belief in the power of authenticity.

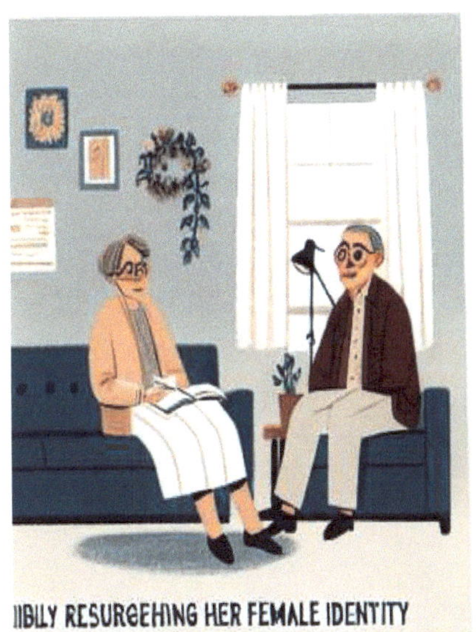
IIBLY RESURGEHING HER FEMALE IDENTITY

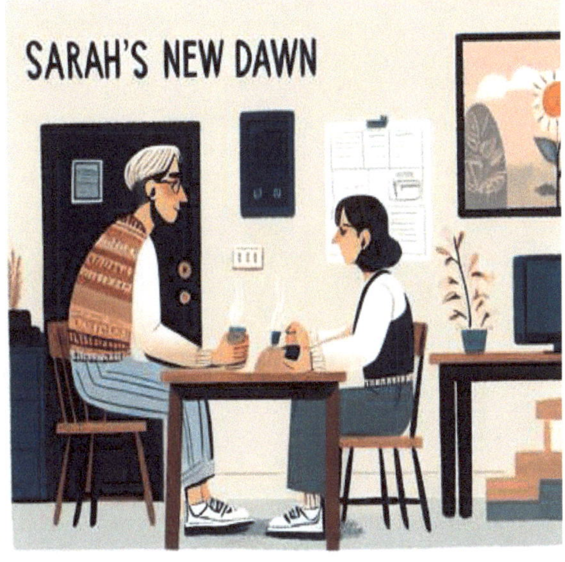
SARAH'S NEW DAWN

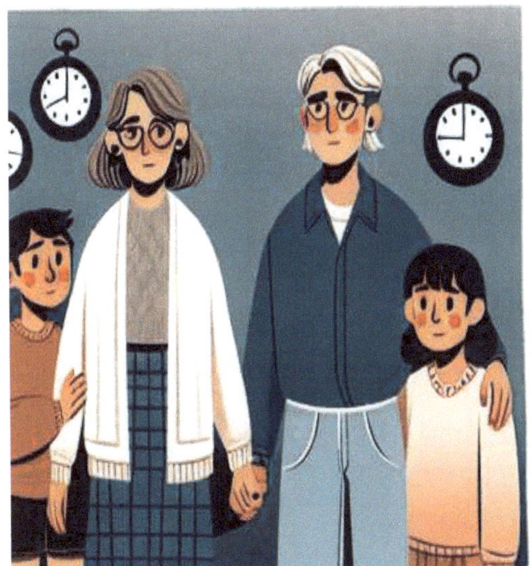
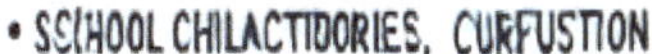
• SCHOOL CHILACTIDORIES, CURFUSTION

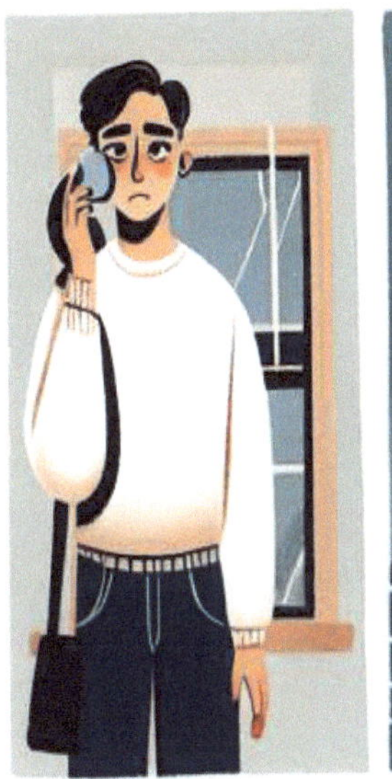
• AA PMIC CHILDREN

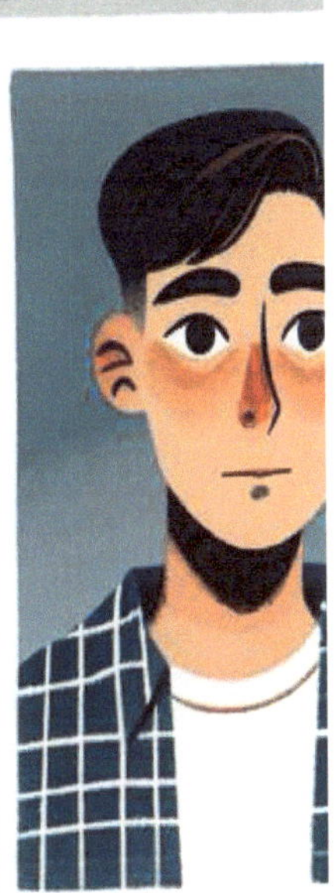
• ASIAN CCN DORAC

Sarah's struggle for acceptance was far from over, but each step forward made the journey worthwhile. She understood now more than ever that acceptance begins within and radiates outward, touching lives in ways unseen but profoundly felt.

3

The Quest for Identity

3.1 Exploring a Dual Existence

Sarah's life took an unexpected turn the morning she woke up to find her reality had shifted in the most profound way imaginable. The physical changes were bewildering enough, but it was the internal turmoil that proved to be the most challenging aspect of her new existence. As she navigated her daily routines, Sarah found herself caught between two identities, each with its own desires, fears, and perspectives.

"How do you feel about all this?" asked Maria, Sarah's closest friend and confidante, over coffee one afternoon. The café buzzed around them, a stark contrast to the intimate bubble of their conversation.

"It's like I'm living two lives," Sarah replied, stirring her coffee absentmindedly. "There's who I was...and who I am now. And they don't fit together easily."

The dialogue between Sarah and Maria opened up avenues for exploring what dual existence meant for Sarah. It wasn't just about gender or physicality; it was about reconciling different parts of oneself in a world that often demands simplicity over complexity.

At work, Sarah faced a different set of challenges. Her colleagues' reactions ranged from supportive to confused to outright hostile. "How do we address you now?" one asked during a particularly tense meeting.

"Just call me Sarah," she responded with a forced smile. "I'm still me." But that interaction highlighted the contradictions of her situation: same yet different, familiar yet unrecognizable.

"Maybe it's not about finding answers," Maria mused towards the end of their conversation. "Maybe it's about learning to live with the questions."

- Navigating personal relationships while adjusting to a new identity

- Dealing with societal expectations and norms

- Finding solace in friendships that offer understanding and support

The journey through dual existence was not just about external acceptance but internal reconciliation. For Sarah, every day brought new questions about identity, belonging, and authenticity. Yet within this tumultuous journey lay opportunities for growth and self-discovery that transcended conventional boundaries.

This insight struck a chord with Sarah. Perhaps embracing her dual existence didn't mean resolving every contradiction but finding peace amidst them. As she left the café that day, Sarah felt a newfound sense of purpose in her complex journey toward self-acceptance.

3.2 Confronting Inner Turmoil

The days following Sarah's realization of her dual existence were marked by a profound inner turmoil. The mirror no longer reflected someone she fully recognized, and the world around her seemed both familiar and utterly alien. It was during one of these tumultuous evenings that Sarah found herself at the doorstep of her brother, Tom, seeking solace in family ties that she hoped remained unaltered.

"I feel like I'm caught in a storm," Sarah confessed as they sat in Tom's dimly lit living room, a space once filled with childhood memories now serving as a backdrop for her adult fears.

"Storms pass," Tom replied gently, his voice a mix of reassurance and uncertainty. "But maybe it's not about waiting for the weather to clear but learning to navigate through it."

This conversation marked the beginning of Sarah's journey into confronting her inner turmoil head-on. With each word exchanged, she delved deeper into the heart of her conflict, articulating feelings that had previously been shapeless shadows in her mind.

- Struggling with the loss of her former self while embracing who she is becoming

- Facing fears of rejection from those unable to understand or accept her transformation

- The challenge of building a bridge between her past and present selves

As the night wore on, Tom shared stories of his own struggles with identity and belonging—a narrative Sarah had only been peripherally aware of. This exchange brought them closer, offering Sarah a glimpse into the universal nature of searching for one's place in the world.

"You're not alone in this," Tom assured her as they parted ways before dawn. "Remember that."

Walking back home under the early morning sky, Sarah felt a shift within herself. The turmoil was still there, but so was a budding sense of clarity and determination. For the first time since her journey began, she felt equipped to face the complexities of her existence—not as insurmountable obstacles but as parts of a larger whole that defined who she was and who she could be.

3.3 Embracing Change

The morning after her profound conversation with Tom, Sarah woke up feeling a mixture of apprehension and excitement. The world outside her window seemed to beckon with a promise of new beginnings. It was in this spirit of hopeful anticipation that she decided to meet with her old friend, Mia, who had always been the epitome of change and adaptation.

"Change is not just about letting go; it's about embracing the new," Mia stated as they walked through the bustling city park, the autumn leaves painting a mosaic of transformation under their feet.

"But how do you embrace something that feels so uncertain?" Sarah asked, watching a leaf detach from its branch and float to the ground.

Mia smiled, "By trusting that you're strong enough to face whatever comes your way. Remember, every leaf falls for a reason, leading to new growth."

This conversation sparked a turning point for Sarah. She began to see her journey not as losing parts of herself but as gaining new depths and dimensions. Her discussions with Mia led to more interactions with others who had navigated their paths through change—each story adding layers to Sarah's understanding and acceptance of her evolving identity.

- Learning to appreciate the beauty in uncertainty
- Finding strength in vulnerability
- Discovering resilience amidst change

As days turned into weeks, Sarah found herself more open to experiences that previously would have daunted her. She started attending workshops on personal growth and even joined a support group for individuals going through significant life transitions.

"You've changed," Tom remarked one evening as they revisited their childhood photo albums.

"I suppose I have," Sarah replied thoughtfully. "But then again, maybe I'm just becoming more myself than ever before."

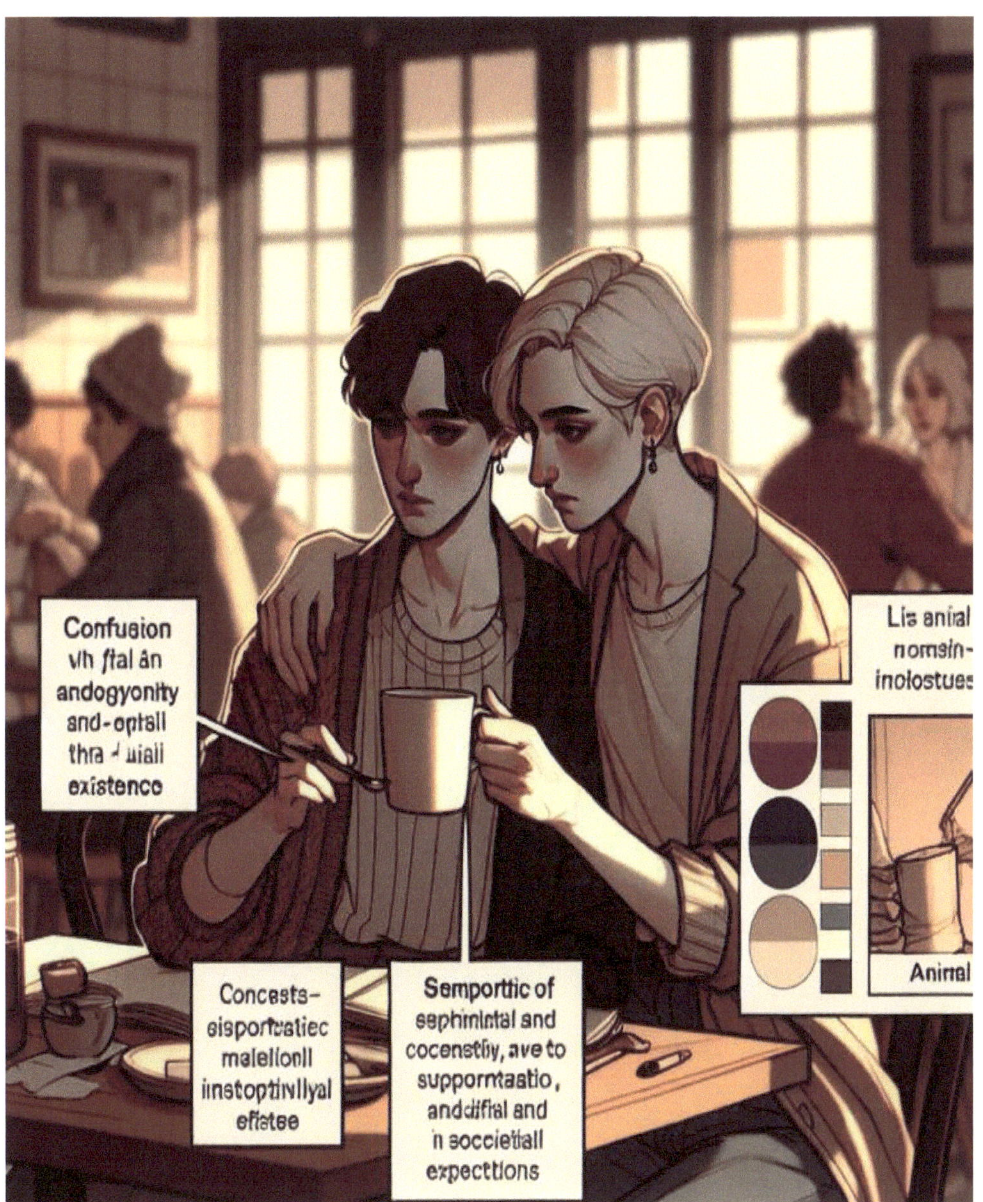

Confusion
vih ftal an
andogyonity
and-optall
thra d uiall
existence
Concosts-
eisporicatiec
malellonll
iinstoptivllyal
efletee
Semportic of
sephimintal and
cocenstly, ave to
supportaatio,
anddifial and
n soccietiall
expecttions
Lia aniral
nomsin-
inolostues
Aniral

Embracing change had not been easy for Sarah, but it had been profoundly rewarding. With each step forward, she felt more aligned with her core self—a self that was continually evolving yet always true. The fear of the unknown still lingered at times, but now it was accompanied by a sense of wonder and possibility.

4

Trials and Tribulations

4.1 Navigating Societal Norms

Sarah, now navigating life with an unexpected transformation, found herself at the crossroads of societal norms and personal identity. The morning after her inexplicable change, she stood before her mirror, a mix of confusion and curiosity painting her features. "How am I supposed to go to work like this?" she muttered to herself, pondering the reactions of her colleagues.

At work, Sarah's new appearance sparked whispers among her coworkers. In a meeting room filled with puzzled glances, she cleared her throat, "I know I look different," she began, seeking understanding in a world that seemed unprepared for such anomalies. Her boss, Mr. Jenkins, adjusted his glasses before speaking up. "We support all our employees here," he said cautiously, "but we also have policies on professional conduct and appearance." Sarah nodded, feeling the weight of societal expectations pressing down on her.

Lunchtime brought an unexpected ally in Lisa, a colleague who had always kept to herself. "I can't pretend to understand what you're going through," Lisa whispered across the table, "but it must be incredibly tough dealing with...all this." Sarah smiled weakly. "You have no idea," she replied. Their conversation meandered from personal struggles to broader issues of gender identity and societal acceptance.

The day ended with Sarah reflecting on her experiences. She realized that navigating societal norms wouldn't be easy but finding community and allies made the path less daunting. As she lay in bed staring at the ceiling, she whispered to herself, "Tomorrow is another day." And with that thought, she drifted off to sleep.

After work, Sarah visited a local support group for transgender individuals recommended by Lisa. There, she met Alex who listened intently to her story. "Society has rigid norms," Alex said thoughtfully after Sarah finished speaking. "But remember, your worth isn't defined by fitting into those boxes." Their words offered comfort but also highlighted the long journey ahead for acceptance and understanding.

4.2 Bonds tested and broken

Sarah's journey through uncharted waters was not without its storms. The days following her transformation saw her relationships with friends and family put to the test, revealing the strength and fragility of bonds once thought unbreakable. "You're just not the person I knew," said Tom, a childhood friend, his words slicing through the air like a cold wind. Sarah's heart sank as she realized that not all would stand by her in this new chapter of her life.

At a family dinner, silence hung heavily over the table after Sarah shared her experiences. Her parents exchanged glances, struggling to bridge the gap between their love for their child and their own ingrained beliefs. "We need time," her mother finally whispered, a statement that felt like an insurmountable distance had been placed between them.

"Why can't you see I'm still me?" Sarah pleaded during a heated conversation with her sister, Emily. Emily paused, tears brimming in her eyes. "I do see you, Sarah. It's just...hard to adjust." This moment of vulnerability marked a turning point, offering a glimmer of hope amidst the turmoil.

The workplace became an arena of its own challenges. While some colleagues like Lisa offered unwavering support, others distanced themselves or cloaked their discomfort in awkward jokes. A project team meeting turned sour when Mark, previously a close work friend, openly questioned Sarah's ability to contribute effectively amidst "all this personal stuff." His words stung with betrayal.

Yet it was within these trials that true allies emerged. Lisa's steadfast friendship provided solace and understanding when Sarah felt most isolated. Together with Alex from the support group, they formed a tight-knit circle that celebrated Sarah for who she was rather than who society expected her to be.

As Sarah navigated these tumultuous waters, she learned valuable lessons about human nature: some bonds may weaken or break under strain but finding those who accept and support you unconditionally paves the way for deeper connections forged in authenticity and mutual respect.

4.3 Finding allies in unexpected places

Sarah's journey, marked by upheaval and transformation, led her down paths she never anticipated. In the wake of strained relationships and lost connections, she discovered solace and support from quarters unforeseen. This chapter unfolds the serendipitous encounters that broadened her circle of allies, enriching her life with new perspectives and unwavering support.

"I never thought I'd find understanding here," Sarah confessed one evening at a local coffee shop to Jenna, the owner who had become an unexpected confidant. Jenna's warm smile over the counter had been the first sign of a budding friendship. "People surprise you," Jenna replied, pouring Sarah's favorite blend. "Sometimes, it's about being in the right place at the right moment."

The narrative took an intriguing turn when Sarah volunteered at a community garden. Here, amidst rows of budding plants, she met Aaron, a retired teacher with a passion for botany and an open heart. "Plants aren't judgmental," he joked one afternoon while showing Sarah how to prune tomatoes properly. "They thrive on care and attention—much like people." His words struck a chord with Sarah, highlighting parallels between nurturing plants and fostering relationships.

Even within her online world, allies emerged from pixels and posts. During late-night browsing sessions on forums dedicated to personal transformation stories, Sarah stumbled upon Maya's blog. Maya's digital diary was filled with tales of resilience and acceptance that resonated deeply with Sarah. A flurry of comments exchanged led to emails, then video calls— a modern friendship rooted in shared experiences.

These newfound connections underscored a vital lesson for Sarah: allies can be found in the most unexpected places, often emerging during times of need. Each encounter served as a reminder that openness to new experiences could lead to meaningful bonds formed on mutual respect and understanding.

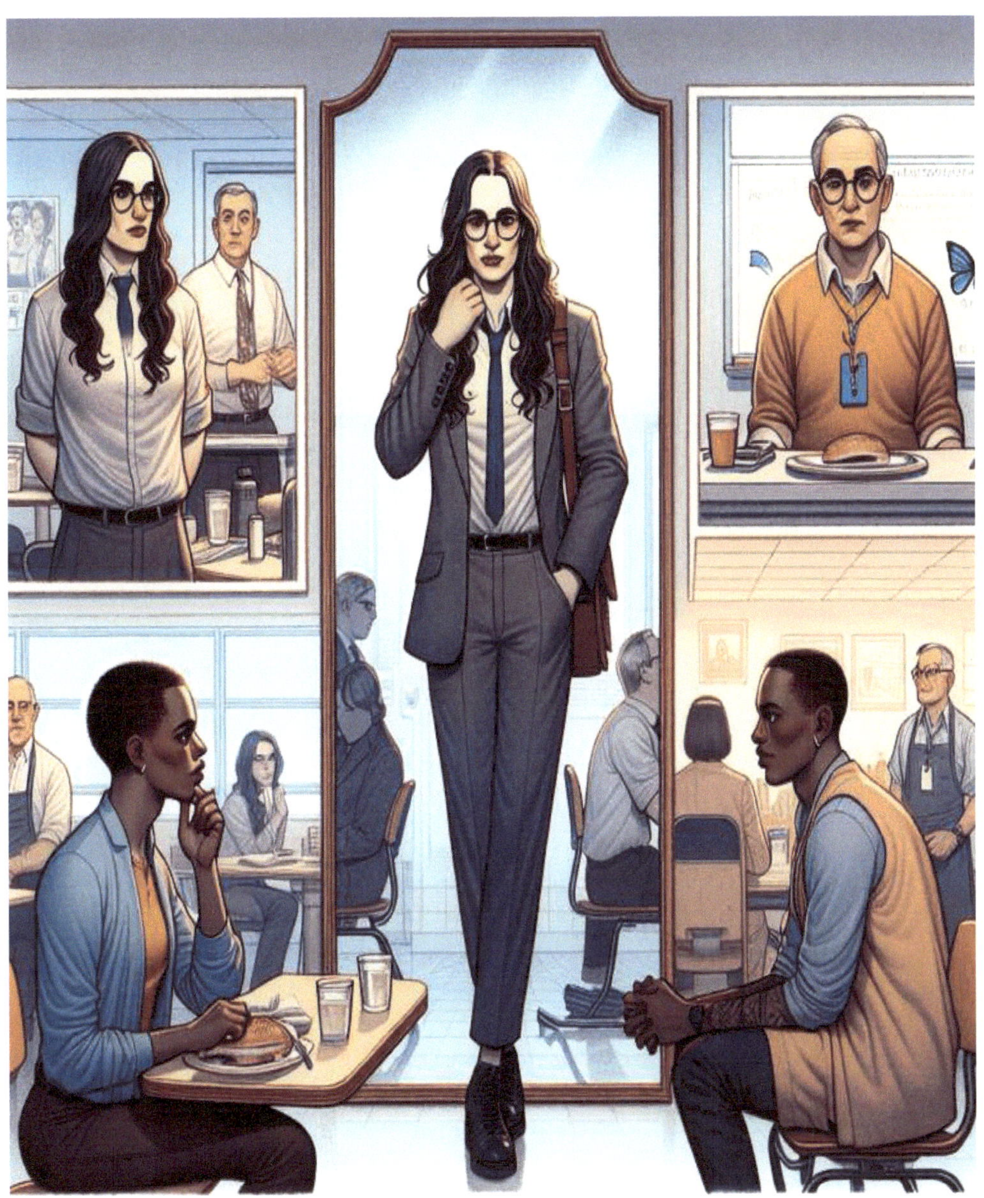

As Sarah reflected on these interactions, she realized that while some doors had closed behind her, others had opened ahead—each leading to opportunities for growth and companionship. Her journey illustrated that even amidst trials, there are always avenues for connection if one remains open to them.

5

The Search for Resolution

5.1 A journey towards understanding

Sarah's life took an unexpected turn the morning she woke up to find her body had undergone a transformation that challenged her understanding of herself and her place in the world. Confused and desperate for answers, she embarked on a journey that would not only test her resilience but also expand her perspective on identity and acceptance.

"I just don't understand how this could happen," Sarah confessed to her closest friend, Jamie, over coffee. The café around them buzzed with the mundane chatter of daily life, a stark contrast to the turmoil brewing within Sarah.

"Maybe it's not about understanding it right away," Jamie suggested gently, "but about accepting yourself as you are now and exploring what this means for you."

Their conversation was interrupted by a stranger at the next table who had overheard their discussion. "Excuse me," he said, "I couldn't help but overhear. You're not alone. There are communities out there who've gone through similar experiences. Maybe they can offer you guidance or support."

This encounter led Sarah to seek out others who had experienced similar transformations or who identified beyond traditional gender binaries. Each person she met offered a new piece of the puzzle, sharing their own stories of confusion, acceptance, and love.

"It's like I'm learning to navigate the world all over again," Sarah admitted during a support group meeting. "But hearing your stories makes me feel less isolated."

Through these interactions, Sarah began to see her situation not as a problem to be fixed but as an opportunity to understand the fluidity of gender and identity more deeply. She realized that while her physical transformation was unexpected, it opened doors to communities and conversations that enriched her view of humanity.

As weeks turned into months, Sarah found strength in her newfound connections. Her journey towards understanding was far from over, but she no longer felt adrift in a sea of confusion. Instead, she embraced her experience as part of a larger narrative of self-discovery and acceptance.

5.2 Challenges of transformation

Sarah's journey of self-discovery was fraught with challenges that tested her resilience at every turn. The initial shock of her transformation had given way to a myriad of emotions, ranging from fear and confusion to a cautious hope for understanding. As she navigated this new reality, the reactions from those around her added layers of complexity to her experience.

"How do you deal with the stares, the whispers?" Sarah asked during one of her meetings with the support group, her voice tinged with frustration.

"It's never easy," replied Alex, a member who had become a close confidant. "But remember, their reactions are more about their own perceptions and less about who you truly are."

Their conversation was punctuated by moments of silence, each person reflecting on their own encounters with societal norms and expectations. It was during these meetings that Sarah found solace in shared experiences, drawing strength from the collective resilience of the group.

Yet, it wasn't just society's gaze that posed a challenge. Sarah grappled with internal conflicts as well. "Some days I look in the mirror and I don't recognize myself," she confessed to Jamie one evening. "It's like I'm caught between who I was and who I'm becoming."

"Transformation isn't just physical, Sarah," Jamie responded softly. "It's also about embracing the changes within you, learning to love yourself anew."

This internal battle was perhaps the most daunting aspect of Sarah's journey. The physical changes were visible for all to see, but the emotional and psychological shifts were hidden battles fought in solitude.

Despite these challenges, Sarah's story is not solely defined by struggle. Each obstacle encountered on her path towards acceptance served as a stepping stone towards greater self-awareness and empathy for others' journeys. Through conversations filled with vulnerability and courage, she slowly began to weave together the fragmented pieces of her identity into a tapestry rich with complexity and beauty.

In facing these challenges head-on, Sarah discovered not only deeper layers of herself but also an unspoken bond that connected her to others walking similar paths. This realization brought comfort during moments of doubt, illuminating her journey with flickers of hope and solidarity.

5.3 Acceptance and the path forward

The journey of acceptance for Sarah was akin to navigating a labyrinth, each turn revealing new truths and challenges. The path forward was illuminated by moments of profound understanding and connection, not only with herself but also with those who had become pillars in her life.

"I think I'm starting to see the light," Sarah shared with Alex during a quiet moment in their favorite café, the hustle of life moving around them. "It's like I'm learning to walk again, but this time, I'm choosing my own direction."

Alex smiled warmly, recognizing the monumental shift in her perspective. "That's all we can ever do, Sarah. Choose our paths and hope they lead us to where we need to be."

This exchange marked a pivotal moment for Sarah. It wasn't about reaching a destination but embracing the journey itself, with all its imperfections and surprises. Her conversations had evolved from seeking answers to sharing insights, a testament to her growth.

Yet acceptance did not mean the absence of struggle. There were days when doubt crept in like an unwelcome shadow, casting long lines across her newfound confidence. It was during these times that Jamie's words became a beacon of hope.

"Remember, transformation is as much about letting go as it is about becoming," Jamie reminded her one evening when the weight of change felt particularly heavy.

Sarah found solace in these words, understanding that acceptance was not a final state but a continuous process of acknowledging her fears and doubts while also celebrating her strengths and victories.

The path forward was lined with lessons learned from each person she encountered on her journey. From Alex's unwavering support to Jamie's gentle wisdom, these relationships forged an unbreakable chain of solidarity that empowered Sarah to move beyond mere acceptance into a realm of genuine self-love and appreciation for life's infinite possibilities.

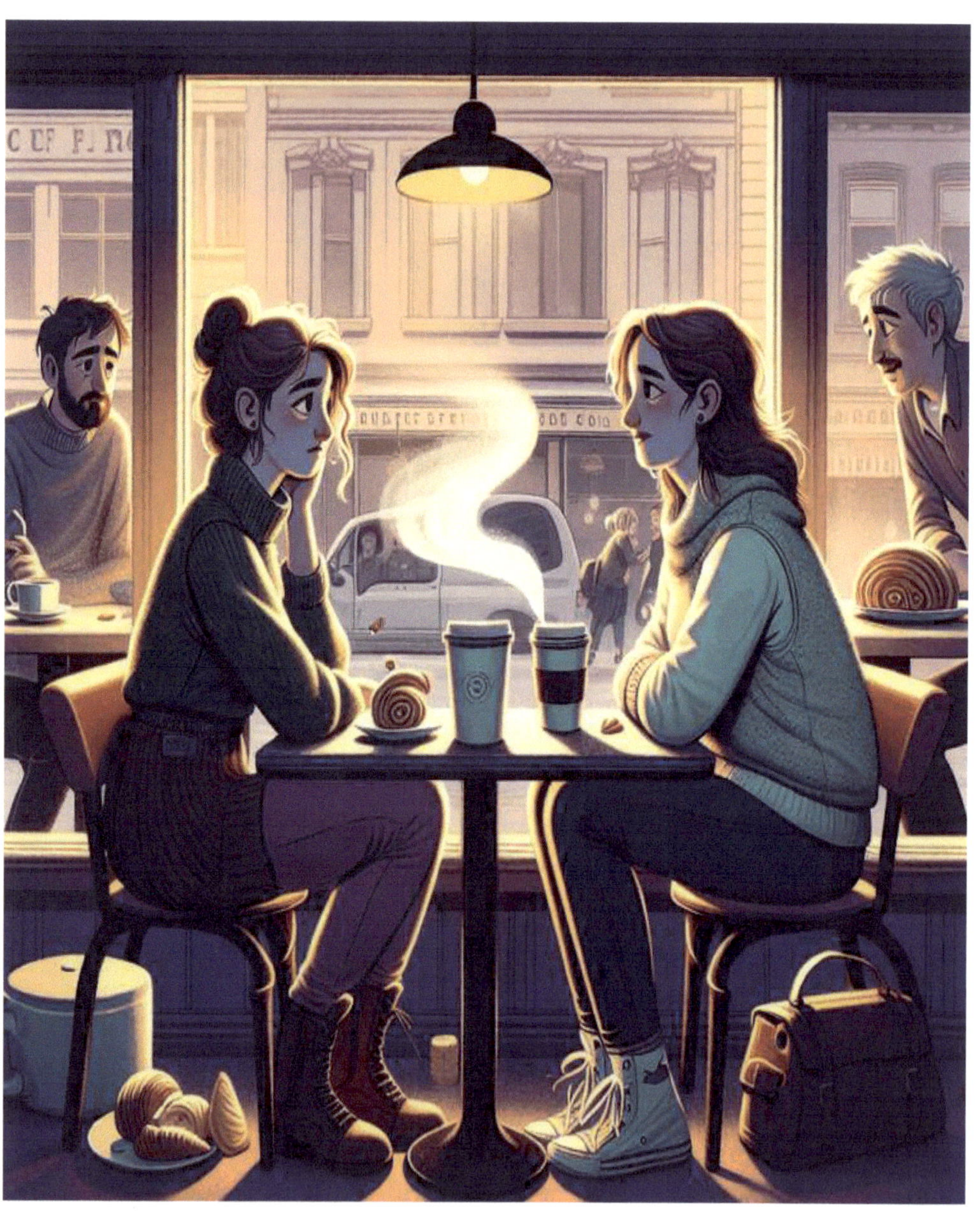

In embracing this journey, Sarah discovered that acceptance was not just about making peace with the changes within herself but also about opening her heart to the world around her. This realization did not signify an end but rather the beginning of a new chapter filled with hope, resilience, and an unyielding spirit ready to face whatever lay ahead.

6

Embracing Change and Moving Forward

6.1 Overcoming Fear and Resistance

Sarah, now facing an unprecedented change in her life, found herself at the crossroads of fear and resistance. The morning light filtered through the curtains, casting a glow on what was now her new reality. She sat at the edge of her bed, grappling with a whirlwind of emotions.

"How am I supposed to face the world like this?" Sarah muttered to herself, her voice a mix of confusion and fear.

Her friend, Jamie, who had been supportive through Sarah's journey of self-discovery and change, noticed the turmoil Sarah was going through. "Sarah," Jamie began gently, "I know this is scary. But maybe it's not about finding immediate answers or solutions. It's about embracing who you are now and moving forward one step at a time."

Sarah sighed deeply, "But what if I can't? What if everyone turns their back on me? My job, my kids... I'm scared of losing everything I've worked so hard for."

Jamie took Sarah's hand in hers, offering a comforting squeeze. "You won't be alone in this. Remember that overcoming fear isn't about eradicating it but facing it with courage. And resistance? It's just another word for an opportunity to grow stronger."

Their conversation was interrupted by a call from Sarah's ex-husband regarding their children. This brought another layer of complexity to her situation but also highlighted the need for open communication and understanding.

"I guess part of overcoming this fear is opening up about it," Sarah pondered aloud after ending the call.

"Exactly," Jamie affirmed. "And remember, resistance often comes from not knowing or understanding. People fear what they can't comprehend. Maybe it's about helping them see beyond traditional norms and expectations."

As the day progressed, Sarah realized that her journey wasn't just about overcoming personal fears but also challenging societal perceptions and barriers. With each conversation she had - whether with family members or colleagues - she felt a piece of the resistance chipping away.

In embracing her new self without succumbing to fear or societal pressures, Sarah discovered an inner strength she never knew existed. It wasn't an easy path by any means; there were moments filled with doubts and setbacks. However, through these experiences, she learned that true courage lies in being authentic to oneself despite the uncertainties ahead.

6.2 Finding Support and Building a Support System

Sarah's journey of self-discovery and change was not one she had to navigate alone. The importance of finding support and building a supportive network became increasingly clear as she faced the challenges ahead. "It's like constructing a bridge while walking on it," Sarah mused during one of her reflective moments.

"You know, Sarah," Jamie said, breaking into her thoughts, "building a support system is crucial. It's about surrounding yourself with people who understand and accept you for who you are." Jamie's words were a beacon of hope in the fog that had enveloped Sarah's mind.

"But how do I even begin?" Sarah asked, feeling overwhelmed by the prospect.

"Start small," Jamie suggested. "Reach out to those closest to you, those you trust implicitly. Then gradually extend your circle to include others who share similar experiences or are open-minded and supportive."

Their conversation led to action. Together, they compiled a list of individuals and groups that could form part of this burgeoning support system:

- Close family members willing to offer emotional support

- Friends like Jamie who provided unwavering encouragement

- Support groups for people undergoing similar life changes

- Mentors or counselors skilled in guiding through transitions

With each person she reached out to, Sarah felt a piece of her isolation fall away, replaced by connections that offered strength and understanding. These interactions varied—some were heartwarming affirmations of unconditional support, while others required patience and time to foster understanding.

"I never realized how many people are willing to stand by me," Sarah reflected after several weeks of slowly building her network.

"And there will be more," Jamie assured her with a smile. "The key is openness—being honest about your needs and fears. It invites others to do the same."

This newfound network did not erase the challenges Sarah faced but provided her with a foundation upon which she could lean during moments of doubt or fear. It was through this tapestry of support that Sarah found not just acceptance but also empowerment—a collective strength that propelled her forward on her journey.

6.3 Setting Goals and Taking Action

Sarah sat across from Jamie, her notebook open to a blank page that seemed as daunting as the journey ahead. "I know I need to set goals, but it feels like standing at the base of a mountain," she confessed, her pen hovering uncertainly.

"Think of it not as one giant leap but a series of steps," Jamie suggested, leaning in. "What's one thing you want to achieve in the near future?"

After a moment of thought, Sarah replied, "I want to be more confident in my decisions." She wrote it down, the first words on the page no longer feeling insurmountable.

"Great start," Jamie smiled. "Now, let's break that down. What actions can take you there?"

Their conversation flowed into action plans:

- Identifying small decisions Sarah could practice with daily

- Finding workshops or books on building confidence

- Setting weekly check-ins with Jamie to reflect on progress and setbacks

With each goal they outlined, Sarah felt a growing sense of direction. It was not just about setting targets but committing to steps that would inch her closer to them.

"And remember," Jamie added, "it's okay if some goals evolve or change. The important thing is that you're moving forward."

This advice struck a chord with Sarah. She realized that flexibility in her approach could be empowering rather than a sign of failure.

As weeks turned into months, Sarah revisited her list often, ticking off achievements and adding new goals. Each small victory bolstered her confidence, not just in decision-making but in her ability to adapt and grow.

"Looking at this list now," Sarah reflected during one of their weekly check-ins, "I see more than just what I've done. I see who I'm becoming."

Jamie nodded, pride evident in their eyes. "And every step you take is proof that you're capable of navigating this journey."

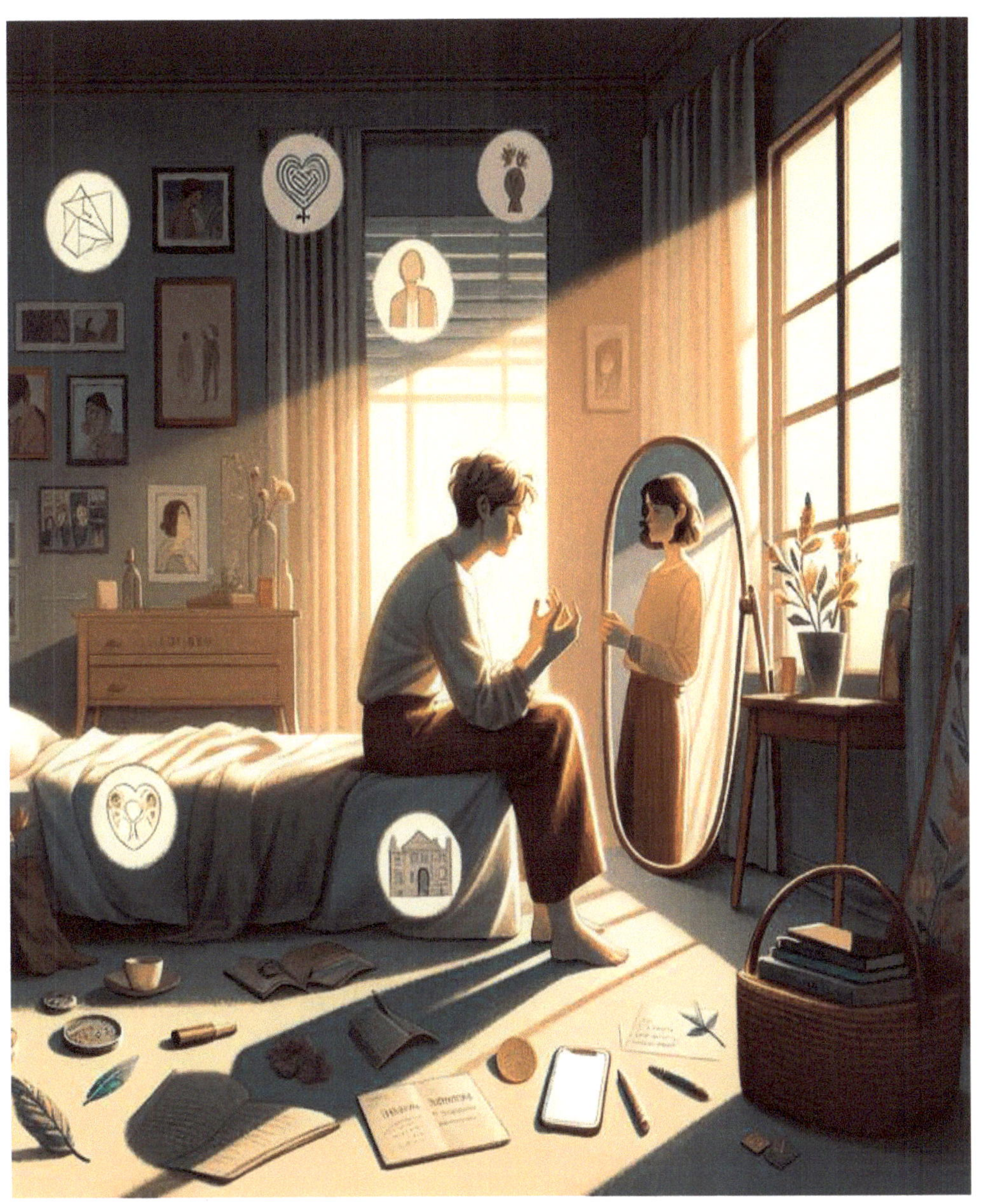

In "If I Was A Man," readers are introduced to Sarah, a single mother grappling with the complexities of life post-divorce. She shares custody of her children with her ex-husband, navigating the challenges that come with co-parenting. Beyond her family struggles, Sarah faces dissatisfaction in her professional life and an overarching sense of discontentment with her existence as a woman.

One morning, Sarah awakens to find herself in an unimaginable situation: she has physically transformed into a man, complete with male genitalia and masculine desires. This shocking change thrusts Sarah into a whirlwind of internal conflict and societal dilemmas. Her newfound male identity brings about a profound crisis, forcing her to confront issues related to gender identity, sexuality, and societal expectations.

As Sarah attempts to navigate her altered reality, she seeks medical advice in hopes of understanding and possibly reversing the transformation. However, the medical community is baffled by her condition, offering no solutions or explanations for her sudden change.

The narrative follows Sarah's journey through this extraordinary circumstance, exploring themes of identity, acceptance, and the fluidity of gender. Through trials and tribulations, Sarah grapples with what it means to live as a man in a world that had always seen her as a woman. The story delves deep into the societal constructs of gender roles and the personal turmoil that arises when those constructs are challenged.

Ultimately, "If I Was A Man" is a thought-provoking exploration of self-discovery against the backdrop of societal norms. It examines how drastically life can shift when one's fundamental identity is altered overnight and how one navigates the path toward understanding oneself amidst unprecedented change. The resolution leaves readers contemplating the essence of identity and the lengths one might go to find peace within themselves.

This synopsis captures the essence of "If I Was A Man," presenting its main plot points while maintaining an air of mystery around how Sarah's journey concludes. It reflects on significant themes without revealing every detail, inviting readers to delve into Sarah's transformative experience firsthand.